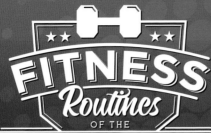

ROGER
FEDERER

JEFF
SAVAGE

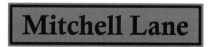

PUBLISHERS

2001 SW 31st Avenue
Hallandale, FL 33009

www.mitchelllane.com

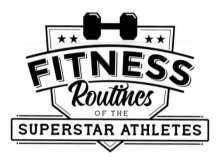

First Edition, 2020.
Author: Jeff Savage
Designer: Ed Morgan
Editor: Lisa Petrillo

Series: Fitness Routines of the Superstar Athletes
Title: Roger Federer / by Jeff Savage

Hallandale, FL : Mitchell Lane Publishers, [2020]

Library bound ISBN: 9781680204650
eBook ISBN: 9781680204667

Contents

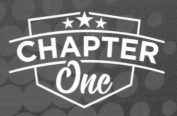

MAKING History

Tennis star Roger Federer was fading. He was playing in the 2018 Australian Open final at Melbourne Park. Entering the title match, the Swiss wizard had steamrolled over his six opponents without dropping a set. In this final contest, he won the first set in a mere 24 minutes. But then his opponent, Marin Cilic, began battling back. The tall Croatian blasted winning shots. Federer struggled to keep up. Two hours later, Federer lost five straight games. The match was tied entering the fifth and final set.

Why was Federer so powerless? Maybe it was the extreme heat. The temperature in Melbourne that day reached 103 degrees Fahrenheit with high **humidity**. After the women's final a day earlier, top-ranked Simona Halep spent the night at the hospital with heat exhaustion. Maybe it was the pressure. Federer was trying to win his sixth Australian Open title. No one in history had won more. "I was thinking about the outcome all day," he admitted afterward. "During the first set, during the second, the third, the fourth. 'How would I feel if I lost? How would I feel if I won?' And it just wouldn't stop."

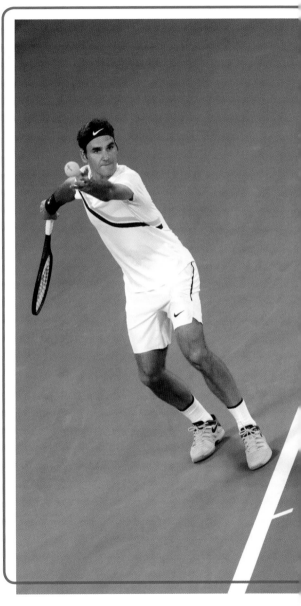

Federer's ace serving was a strength at the 2018 Australian Open.

Chapter ONE

Or maybe it was his age. At 36, Federer was considered an "old" player. Nearly all tennis players retire well before then. Federer was trying to become the oldest winner of a **Grand Slam** tournament in 45 years.

Federer sat on a bench along the blue court to prepare for the final grueling set. The packed crowd at Rod Laver Arena watched him closely. Federer drank from his sports bottle and wiped a towel across the back of his neck. Rod Laver himself, for whom the arena was named, sat in the front row, snapping pictures of Federer with his phone. Laver was the greatest Australian tennis player ever. He retired long ago and never played against Federer. But Laver knew him well. In 2006, he presented Federer with the winner's trophy, as Federer cried with joy. In 2017, just a year earlier, he did so again, and Federer wept again. This time, Laver knew Federer was drained. But he also knew Federer wasn't done. "He's playing as well as he did 10 years ago," Laver had told reporters when the tournament started. "He's playing smarter. He sees weaknesses in his opponents that other people can't see. That's the difference between Roger and everyone else."

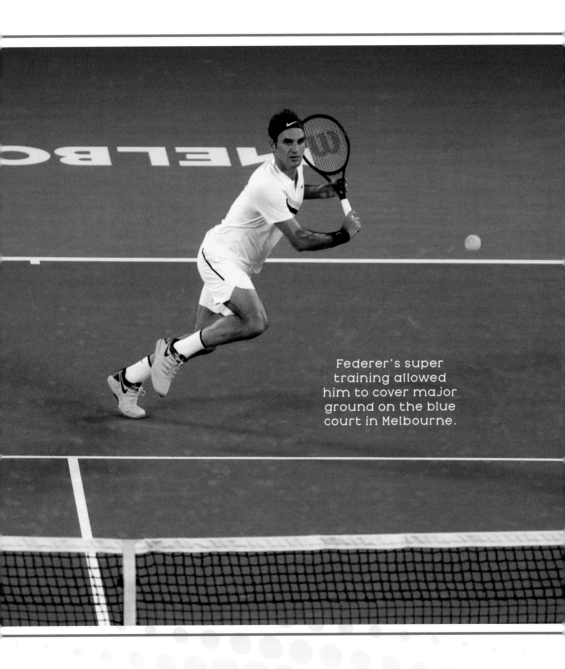

Federer's super training allowed him to cover major ground on the blue court in Melbourne.

Federer opened the fifth set with force. He smashed serves past Cilic. He ripped forehands crosscourt and chipped backhands neatly into corners. He played with joy and ease, almost seeming to float weightless on the court. Cilic was helpless. In the final game, Federer hammered an ace, forced Cilic into two misses, and slammed home one last ace to win 6-1 and make history. How was this possible?

Federer received the trophy and sobbed again. "It's a dream come true and the fairy tale continues," he said to the crowd. "It's incredible. I've won three Slams in 12 months. I can't believe it myself."

Fun Fact

Roger was a ball boy at his hometown tennis tournament in Basel, Switzerland. His favorite part was getting a pizza party with the champion. As a pro, Federer has won the Basel tournament nine times. His favorite part is the pizza party with the ball kids.

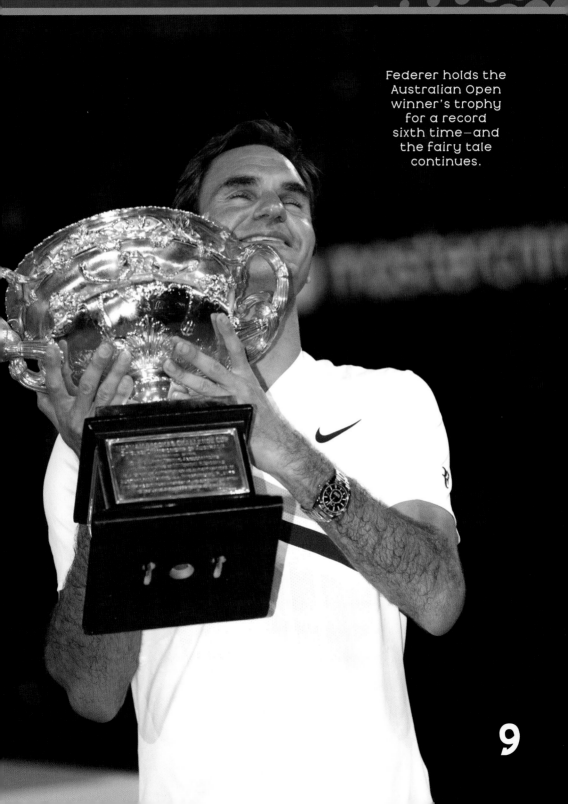

Federer holds the Australian Open winner's trophy for a record sixth time—and the fairy tale continues.

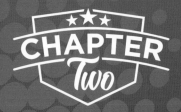

CHAPTER Two

Reaching the TOP

Roger Federer was born August 8, 1981, in Basel, Switzerland. His parents, Robert and Lynette, raised him and his older sister, Diana. Roger was 4 years old when he got his first tennis racket. He raced around the house hitting balls off bedroom walls and kitchen cabinets. "He had to keep moving." his mother said. "Otherwise he became unbearable."

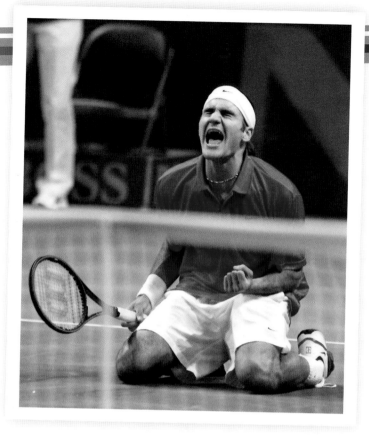

Federer has always poured out his emotions on the court.

Roger played tennis regularly by age 6, joined a local club at 8, and began private lessons at 10. He enjoyed the subject math in school, played the piano, and participated in other sports like basketball, badminton, and soccer. But at age 12 he knew he wanted to become a professional athlete, and so he decided to drop everything else and choose one sport. "I enjoyed the position I was in as a tennis player," he explained to a magazine writer. "With tennis, I was to blame when I lost. I was to blame when I won. I really liked that because I played a lot of soccer too, and I couldn't stand it when I had to blame it on the goalkeeper."

Roger left home at age 13 for Switzerland's national tennis training center. He practiced the sport and attended school and returned home on weekends by train. At first he was homesick, crying Sunday nights as he rode the train two hours back to the center. Eventually he adjusted and thrived.

At age 17 he won the Junior Wimbledon title. In 1999 Federer joined the Association of Tennis Professionals (ATP Tour), and four years later he became the first Swiss ever to win a Grand Slam when he captured the Wimbledon championship. He dominated men's tennis after that, winning five straight Wimbledon titles and five straight U.S. Open crowns.

Entering 2019, he has appeared in 30 slam finals and won 20 of them—both all-time records. At a tournament in 2018, he regained the world No. 1 ranking at age 36, becoming the oldest player to do so. "This maybe means the most to me in my career," Federer told the crowd. "At the beginning you kind of get there because you played so well, but later in your career you have to fight for it and wrestle it back from someone. You have to put double the work in."

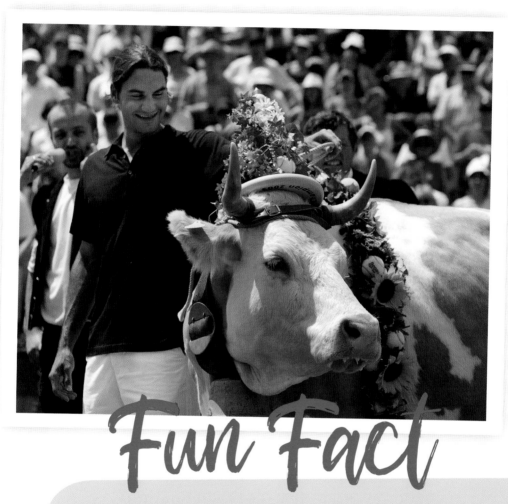

Fun Fact

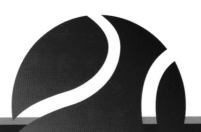

At the 2003 Swiss Open, Federer was given a gift for winning Wimbledon one week earlier. A milking cow! He named her Juliette.

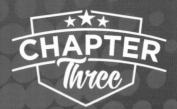

CHAPTER
Three

Smart
TRAINING

Tennis is a physically demanding sport. Players scamper around the court, stressing their muscles and joints. Injuries happen. A player forced to withdraw due to injury is said to "retire" from the match. Roger Federer's toughest rivals have retired many times. For instance, Rafael Nadal and Pete Sampras have retired seven times each, Novak Djokovic and Andre Agassi 11 times each. Federer has *never* retired from a match. How can this be?

Federer conditions his body with intense fitness training. He is so smart that some years he doesn't have a regular coach. "I think there is a benefit to figuring things out for myself," he told a reporter. "I don't need to sit down with a coach and talk about an opponent for an hour. It takes me basically 15 seconds to come up with a game plan. I know everything I need to know." But Federer has always had a fitness trainer—Pierre Paganini. Federer hired Paganini when he joined the pro tour and has been with him ever since.

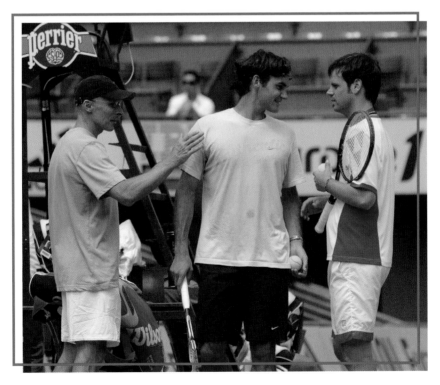

Fitness trainer Pierre Paganini (*left*) and practice coach Severin Luthi (*right*) help Federer with his conditioning.

Federer works with Paganini in Switzerland or Dubai, a city in the Middle East. Paganini rarely travels to tournaments. He has been with Federer for just two of his 20 major wins. When Federer is not on tour, he is with Paganini, fine-tuning his body like a high-performance engine. What do they work on? Everything. Most players have one style and hit the same type of shots repeatedly.

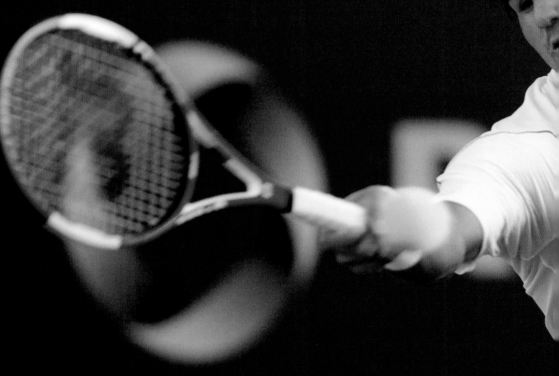

Federer frustrates opponents with his ability to hit all types of shots.

Federer has assorted styles and hits an array of smashes, slices, chips, and drops. He has invented shots that are named for him. He bounces around the court like a giant spring. Paganini calls Federer's style "coordinated creativity." For Federer to compete this way, he must perform challenging exercises for **agility**, coordination, balance, reaction time, strength, and **endurance**.

Federer warms up by jumping rope, jogging around the court, and **shuffling** from side to side. After several minutes he is ready to go. For agility, he puts a **resistance band** around his legs and moves around the court hitting shots. Then he wraps the band around his waist and connects the other end to the net and plays more that way. For coordination, he places three cones in a triangle near the baseline and zigzags between them while hitting shots. For balance, he stands on a mini-trampoline and hits **volleys**. Then he stands on one leg and hits more. For reaction time, his trainer throws three balls to him at the same time from about 10 feet away. He quickly hits each ball, one at a time, before they bounce a second time.

Federer focuses heavily on strength. He works his core, or midsection, by performing several exercises. He does lateral lunges by placing a barbell across his shoulders, stepping forward and down, and twisting his upper body in a motion similar to hitting a forehand or backhand. This exercise converts to great shot power on the court.

He tosses a **medicine ball** back and forth to his trainer across the net as he **shuffles** from sideline to sideline. He performs other basic core exercises such as **leg raises** and **crunches**. Federer is 6 feet 1 inch tall, and weighs 177 pounds. He has a narrow waist and muscular shoulders. In the weight room he does bench presses, **flys**, **pull-downs**, and curls. He does not like to do pushups. Paganini makes him do them anyway.

Novak Djokovic (*background*) marvels at Federer's fitness while watching his rival perform perfect pushups before a match.

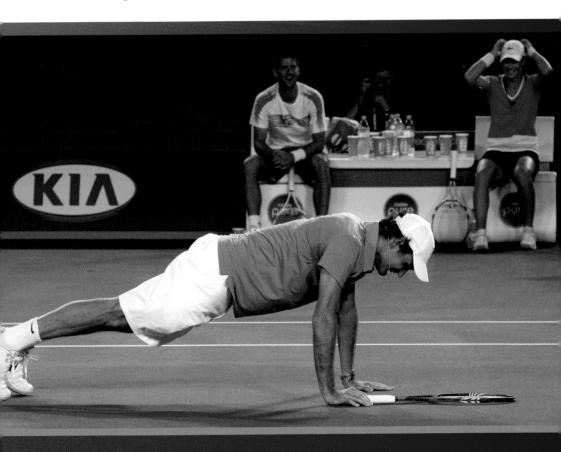

For endurance, Federer does a grueling jump rope workout. He skips for 60 seconds, drops the rope, and performs a 60-second **plank**. He skips for another 60 seconds, then does side planks. Back and forth he goes, from the rope to exercises, working his core and upper body. He does single and double skips with the rope. This workout lasts about half an hour and leaves him breathless. "You have to put in the effort," Federer told a magazine writer. "A big part of the reason that I am where I am today is definitely because of Pierre. He has made fitness workouts so enjoyable, if they ever can be. I just follow his beat. Whatever he tells me to do, I do it because I trust him."

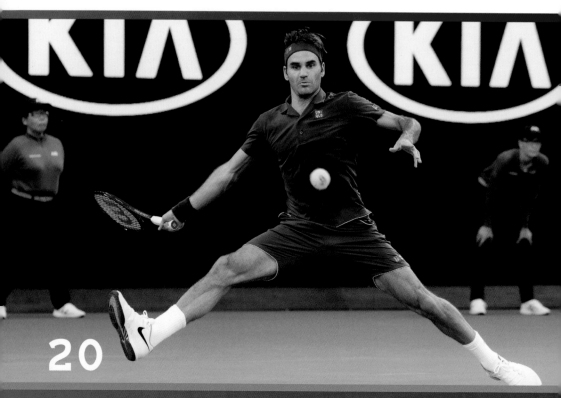

Federer thrills the crowd in Melbourne again as he dominates at the 2019 Australian Open.

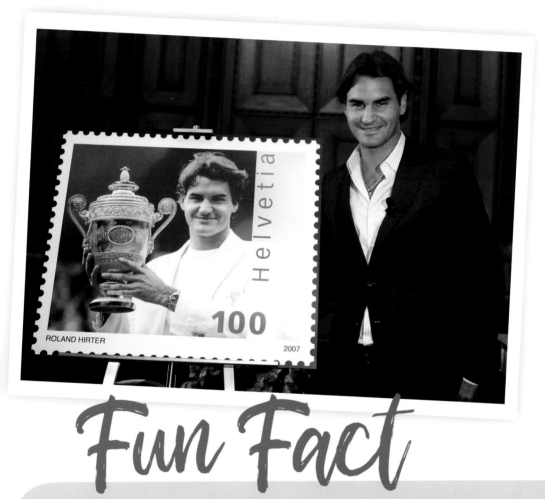

Fun Fact

Federer became the first living Swiss person to be featured on a Switzerland postage stamp. He is pictured holding up the Wimbledon champion trophy.

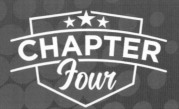

CHAPTER Four

POSITIVE Health

Federer maintains his fitness by eating healthy foods. He eats carbohydrates, fruits, and vegetables for energy, as well as plenty of protein to build muscle. What he eats, and when he eats, depends on whether he is playing a match that day.

On a competition day, Federer watches the clock. Exactly two hours before his match begins, he eats a full plate of pasta with a light sauce. This has been his routine for more than 20 years. Pasta is a slow-burning food that provides fuel for hours. But Federer is not finished fueling his body. He burns approximately 600 calories per hour during a match.

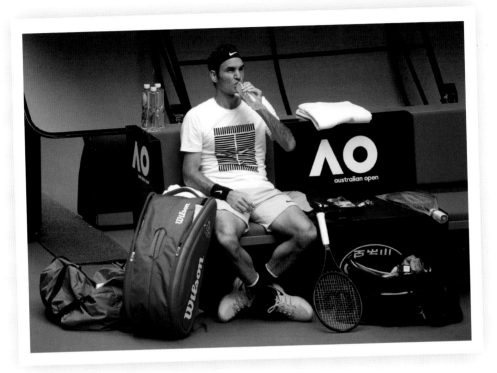

Federer gives his body energy during a match by drinking up to a gallon of fluids and eating healthy snacks.

Federer's matches can last three hours or more. His body needs more energy. On the bench during changeovers, he refuels with healthy snack bars and energy drinks. He sweats so much that he consumes up to a gallon of fluids to stay hydrated. He also eats bananas, because they provide potassium to help prevent cramping. To recover immediately after a match, he eats a meal of carbohydrates and proteins.

On non-match days, Federer is not so strict. For breakfast he enjoys homemade waffles with fresh fruit. He drinks juice and coffee. He takes a shot of apple cider vinegar for its potential health benefits. During the day he eats lean protein, rice and pasta, and salads. After workouts he drinks protein shakes with fruit. He enjoys eating dinner at restaurants. Italian, Japanese, and Indian food are his favorites. He does not turn down desserts. "It's a way to enjoy life," he explained. "I like my ice cream. I like my chocolate. I like my treats. I don't feel bad about it. I can do it and stay in shape for tennis at the same time."

Tennis is a mental sport. A player is either standing on the court or sitting on the bench resting—alone with his thoughts—for hours. When things aren't going well, doubt and frustration can take over. As a teenager, Roger allowed negative thoughts to consume him. He screamed at himself, threw balls out of the court, and smashed his racket. Looking back, he called such behavior "horrible." But as he grew older, he worked hard to change his outlook. He learned to think good thoughts.

Now when he struggles, he uses his mental training. He thinks of past victories. He imagines hitting his next shot for a winner. He visualizes holding up a trophy. He still gets emotional, like when he cries after winning big matches. But he is always training his mind to stay positive. "Every match is physical and mental," he told a magazine writer. "I used to think it was just technique, but it's more. I try to push myself to not get upset and to stay positive. That's been my biggest improvement over all these years. I'm a very positive thinker now. That is what helps me the most in difficult moments."

Fun Fact

Federer speaks four languages—German, Swiss German, English, and French.

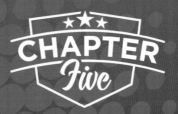

GIVING Back

R oger Federer is adored worldwide. In 2016, he was voted Fan Favorite of the ATP pro tour— *for the 14th straight year!* In a 2011 poll, he was voted the second most respected and admired personality in the world behind human rights icon Nelson Mandela. Federer remains humble. "It's nice to be important," he told a reporter. "But it's more important to be nice."

When Federer became a professional tennis player, his father advised him to try to reach the Top 100 in order to make enough money to earn a living. Federer has done more than that.

The leading finance magazine *Forbes* recently named Federer "the world's most valuable sports brand." He earns several million dollars each year in prize money and many millions more in **endorsements** from companies that sell cars, jewelry, sporting goods, and other products. Federer's estimated worth is half a billion dollars.

Federer is generous with his money. The Roger Federer Foundation has spent more than $30 million for schools and educational programs in Africa. Federer gives millions more to provide food and clothing to the needy all over the world. He plays **exhibition** matches against other highly ranked players to raise millions for charity. He spends as much time as possible with his wife, Mirka, and his four children—identical twin girls Myla and Charlene, and identical twin boys Leo and Lenny. Finally, of course, he devotes time to tennis.

"When you're good at something, make that everything," Federer explained. "You have to put in a lot of sacrifice. There is no way around the hard work. But if you put in the right effort, the reward will come. I can't stay No. 1 for fifty years, you know. But when you do something best in life, you don't really want to give that up—and for me, that's tennis."

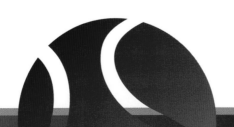

AWARDS

Australian Open Champion
6 times (2004, 2006, 2007, 2010, 2017, 2018)

French Open Champion
1 time (2009)

Wimbledon Champion
8 times (2003, 2004, 2005, 2006, 2007, 2009, 2012, 2017)

U.S. Open Champion
5 times (2004, 2005, 2006, 2007, 2008)

Sportsman of the Year (Laureus)
5 times (2005, 2006, 2007, 2008, 2018)

ATP Player of the Year
5 times (2004, 2005, 2006, 2007, 2009)

ITF (International Tennis Federation) Player of the Year
5 times (2004, 2005, 2006, 2007, 2009)

TIMELINE

1981 — born in Basel, Switzerland

1998 — won Junior Wimbledon

1998 — named world champion

1999 — began competing on the ATP Tour

2003 — won first Wimbledon title (first Grand Slam title)

2004 — won first Australian Open title

2004 — won first U.S. Open title

2007 — won fifth consecutive Wimbledon title

2008 — won fifth consecutive U.S. Open title

2009 — won first French Open title

2017 — won eighth Wimbledon title

2018 — won sixth Australian Open title

GLOSSARY

agility   The ability to move quickly and easily

crunches   Exercise in which you lie on your back with your knees bent and feet flat on the floor and raise your upper body slightly off the floor while holding in your stomach

endorsement   Money paid by a company to someone in exchange for promoting its product

endurance   The ability to remain active for a long period of time without tiring out

exhibition   A tennis match that is not played as part of a tournament

flys   Exercise in which you hold a weight in either hand with arms straight and bring your hands together

grand slam   One of four major tournaments held each year (Australian Open, French Open, Wimbledon, U.S. Open)

humidity   The amount of water vapor in the air

leg raises   Exercise in which you lie on your back with legs extended and slowly raise and lower your legs

medicine ball   A ball usually the size of a basketball but much heavier

plank   Exercise in which you hold steady in a pushup position

pull-downs   Exercise performed on a pulley machine in which you grab a bar overhead at either end and pull it down to neck or chest level

resistance band   Ropes made of rubber or latex that stretch like big rubber bands, some with a handle at both ends

shuffles   Exercise from a crouched position in which you step sideways with one foot and then the other without crossing feet

volley   Shot hit out of the air before it bounces

FURTHER READING

Brown, Anne K. *Roger Federer*. Detroit: Lucent
  Books, 2012.

Glaser, Jason. *Roger Federer*. New York: Gareth
  Stevens, 2012.

Savage, Jeff. *Roger Federer*. Minneapolis: Lerner
  Publications, 2009.

ON THE INTERNET

www.rogerfederer.com
Federer's official site

www.atpworldtour.com
Association of Tennis Professionals official site

www.itftennis.com
International Tennis Federation official site

INDEX

ABOUT the AUTHOR

Jeff Savage is the award-winning author of more than 200 books for young readers. A former sportswriter for the *San Diego Union-Tribune*, Jeff's books have been read by millions. Jeff lives with his wife, Nancy, sons Taylor and Bailey, and dogs Tunes, Coach, Ace, Champ, Tank, and Lexi (that's six!) in Folsom, California. Jeff owns three tennis rackets. Comparisons with Roger Federer end there.